The Celebrity's Guide to *Medical Security*

Copyright Lance Hodge, 2016

ISBN-13: 978-1532911903

Printed in the United States of America

Updated: 9/20

I mentioned on the back cover of this book that I began writing this the day after Prince died. If that event had not happened, I probably would not have been motivated to write this book. I imagine that celebrity deaths are not happening at some increased rate, but it sure seems like it. And then, later, Tom Petty died. The story repeats itself every day, people die. The story isn't usually news, but a celebrity death, well, we all hear about that, *that* makes the news. Some of these deaths could have been prevented!

Through their acting, or their music, or their creativity in some realm of business, these celebrities have touched many of us. We may feel we know them somehow. They often affect our lives, and sometimes profoundly. I wasn't a huge Prince fan, but now, after all the news coverage, I realize I missed a lot, and that Prince was remarkable in so many ways.

Too often the story involves drugs. My focus here is not only that, it is the unforeseen medical emergency, whatever the cause. For the high-profile person there is often an ability that most of us don't have, the ability to afford a staff, to have people around them who serve as personal security perhaps. This book is my attempt to make the case for *Medical Security.*

Lance Hodge

THE CELEBRITY'S GUIDE TO
MEDICAL SECURITY

By Lance Hodge, Paramedic

Note to the rich and famous:

If you are a celebrity, or anyone who has people around you to provide some level of security, and you've come across this book somehow, well, you should read it, at least the first chapter. You might think the people around you *are* prepared to act in the event of a medical emergency, maybe you require them to be CPR certified; well that's not good enough. In the first few pages, I hope I can make the case that you should have well-trained *Medical Security*. So take a few minutes, read the first chapter, it's only a few pages. See if I make my case.

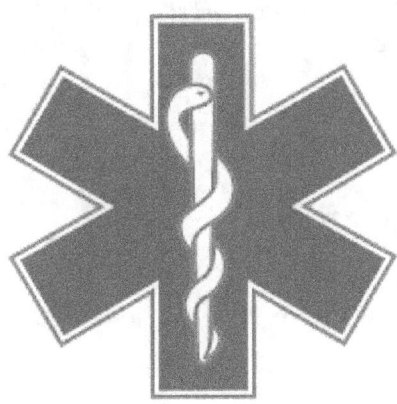

Celebrity: A widely known or famous person.

~

Although the book's title is about "celebrity," I mean more than that. If we all had the means, we might choose to train numerous people around us in important life-saving skills, so that they could help **us** in the event of a potentially life-threatening medical emergency. For those who can do that, this is about you, "celebrity" or not.

~

Note:
I'll use the term "celebrity" often in this book, but it could be "high-profile" or "client" or "person." When it comes to medical emergencies, there is no dividing line, we are all vulnerable, we are all people, together here on this little blue planet, and we all matter. As you'll see on the last page, my focus is two-fold, one; this "business" of training the high-profile client, and two; a commitment to get more AED's placed in more public places and homes.

Chapter One

"BE PREPARED"

The Boy Scouts have a good motto,
"Be prepared."

Medical Security is mostly overlooked by those who put significant effort into *other* security measures. *Medical Security* insures that in the event you, a family member, or someone close to you has a sudden medical emergency there is someone immediately present who can intervene quickly and appropriately to render emergency medical care, until other resources arrive.

The celebrity often has no problem accepting the fact that their *physical* security is important, but what about their *Medical Security*? Too often their *medical* well-being isn't given the same attention. *This mistake has been fatal...*

Prince, Michael Jackson, Amy Winehouse, John Belushi, Jimi Hendrix, Marilyn Monroe, Janis Joplin, Philip Seymour Hoffman, Jim Morrison, James Gandolfini, Tom Petty, and the list goes on and on. *(That's a depressing list!)*

Note: Most often, the people closest to us don't know what to do and are not prepared to act quickly and appropriately in a medical emergency. Most of us don't have that training. Proper training can make the difference between life and death.

~

There are medical conditions so extreme or so damaging that they *will* be fatal, and perhaps *nothing* can be done to save the victim, but, often, with rapid and appropriate medical care, a life may be saved. This is especially true with drug overdose emergencies but is equally important for other medical conditions that might occur. Sometimes just *breathing* for the victim can save them. Sometimes the administration of a simple 'antidote' for a narcotic overdose will revive the victim, but these actions must happen quickly, by someone present near the scene when the emergency occurs, hopefully by someone in the person's immediate circle. Unless proper first aid is given within *the first few minutes*, it may be too late to save them. Calling 9-1-1 for help is NOT enough!

This concept of *Medical Security* must be thought of in terms of personal protection, like a bodyguard. The *Medical Security* personnel are even more 'personal' than the bodyguard. Take the case of Michael Jackson. He was attended by a *highly* paid personal physician, who left Michael unwatched long enough that his breathing stopped, then his heart, and then he died. If Michael had had a Medical Security person at his side, that person could have detected a breathing problem, intervened themselves to breathe for Michael, and of course would have alerted the distracted Doctor to the condition. *Medical Security*, if immediately present, can be lifesavers.

Most often celebrities have some sort of *entourage*. Sometimes large, sometimes obvious, sometimes small, and sometimes discrete, but there is most often *some* inner circle surrounding the rich and famous. Often, this entourage does NOT include someone with *significant* emergency medical training.

The list that began this chapter was depressing, we have lost too many of our gifted artists, most at too young an age. Some of those deaths could probably have been prevented, or at the very least have been given a fair chance at survival with the prompt and appropriate application of medical intervention. Calling 9-1-1, as we'll soon demonstrate, isn't enough. If a burglar enters your home and you have no method of self-defense and that person is intent on harming you, and all you do is call 9-1-1, well, the police will arrive, but their service to you may be the drawing of a chalk line around your body, and a nice investigation that *might* catch your killer. But YOU wouldn't be very pleased with *that* outcome. If you are the victim of a *medical emergency*, you need someone **right there, right now**, who can provide you with the proper emergency medical intervention that might save your life. **Only** calling 9-1-1, well, we don't like chalk outlines, or a ride to the coroner's office, that's a bad day.

Too often when people don't know what to do, they may panic, and calling 9-1-1 may be *all* they do.

It is often the application of quick and appropriate medical first aid by someone *immediately at the scene* that can make the difference between life and death.

Calling 9-1-1 is *vitally* important, but when time is critical, and a life hangs in the balance, it is also vital that someone *at the scene* knows what to do RIGHT NOW *before* help arrives. If breathing stops for more than just a few minutes the heart will stop. If the heart stops for more than just a few minutes the brain will die, and *that* is permanent. *(Brain death is virtually assured if the brain is deprived of oxygen for **more than 4-6 minutes!**)*

The clock is ticking…

Someone collapses. Maybe they've stopped breathing. Maybe their heart has stopped. Nobody at the scene knows for sure what's happened, there's confusion, and panic. Someone says, "Call 9-1-1!" Hopefully that decision to call for help was made *quickly*, and hopefully they didn't call someone else first, to ask *them* what to do; hopefully they didn't call the person's doctor, who would most likely say, "Call 9-1-1!" If we're lucky, the call is placed within **30 seconds** of the time the person collapsed, if we're lucky. Then a dispatcher must ask several important questions. This might take **one minute**. The dispatcher must then activate the closest emergency units to respond and relay the information about the problem and give the address. Let's say that took them **30 seconds**. The responders get the information and respond quickly, let's say in **60 seconds** they are in route to the call. Depending on how far away they are the response time could be significant, and remember this clock keeps ticking. Let's just say the response time to the location is **three and a half minutes**, it would likely be *significantly* longer than that. The rescuers arrive, they gather their equipment and walk to the location. We'll say that took **30 seconds.** They enter the location and quickly assess the victim. That takes maybe **20 seconds.** Then, finally, they administer potential life-saving care.

I've got a calculator…

That's 7 minutes and 30 seconds, to get potential life-saving treatment, *if* everything works just right, *if* the call is made right away, *if* there's no traffic, *if* there's no delay walking up the stairs or taking an elevator or encountering a locked gate, etc. More than seven minutes from the time someone has stopped breathing or their heart has stopped. **More than seven minutes**, *if* everything goes *just right*. Irreversible brain death occurs after **4-6 minutes**. *Houston, we have a problem.*

This book is intended as a general guide, and a text to accompany a *Medical Security Team Training class*. This message, and the point of this little book, is for those people who can afford to add an extra level of protection to their lives. Potential risks and hazards to our well-being are very real. We've seen what has happened to others in the news, but we can improve *our* chances, by training those around us. **We need to make *Medical Security* a priority.**

I'm a Paramedic. I handled more than 15,000 9-1-1 calls as a *Los Angeles City Fire Department* Paramedic. I've been a college EMT (Emergency Medical Technician) instructor for many years and have taught *thousands* of EMT students. I'm a former Reserve L.A. County Sheriff's Deputy and Sheriff's Search and Rescue Team member. I may not have 'seen it all' but I've seen a LOT.

Often our mortality isn't apparent to us, most of us don't *deal* with death, and unless we are quite old we expect to be around for a long time. But life happens, or, as a wise philosopher once said, "Shit happens."

As a Fire Department Paramedic in a big city I dealt with the aftermath of accidents and unexpected medical problems. I administered an antidote for Heroin (opioid) overdoses and brought people back from the brink of death. A *few minutes* made the difference; if we had arrived just a few minutes later they would have had no chance. If we got there 'in time' they would live. It was often black and white, live or die, and the deciding factor was "Time."

The whole point of this book, the essence of it, is the realization that we might be able to survive a serious medical emergency if help arrives *in time*. We may not have to die, now.

As I outlined a few pages ago, the professional help that will arrive when we call 9-1-1 is likely to arrive *too late*. It is the nature of *time* and *physiology* in a medical emergency, not necessarily a defect in the medical response system, as we calculated earlier.

If I make my case here, perhaps more of those with the means will improve their *Medical Security*, they will institute a training program so that their staff and loved ones can better respond to a medical emergency. If properly trained Medical Security is on staff and at the scene, the proper help will arrive *in time*; that is my hope.

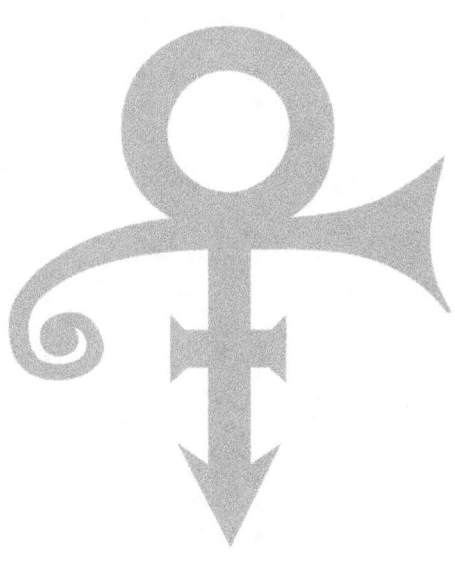

Chapter Two

MEDICAL SECURITY:
WHAT WE DO

Quick medical intervention from trained bystanders, in this case a member of the *Medical Security Team*, plus more advanced intervention by EMT's and Paramedics, and quick transport for definitive hospital care, are THE keys to surviving a serious medical emergency.

Heart attack, stroke, breathing problems, fainting, bleeding, broken bones, seizures, allergic reactions, drug overdoses, choking, and more… we MUST have people around us who are trained in basic first aid for such emergencies. We need trained *Medical Security* who can act quickly, respond calmly, and who can maintain basic life functions for the victim while they await the arrival of 9-1-1 resources.

Our *Medical Security* is as important, maybe *more* important than just physical security. The *Medical Security* I'm discussing in this book doesn't require hiring anyone new. People already on staff can be trained. *Medical Security* can become another aspect of their job for someone already on the payroll. The cost of training such persons is relatively small, and this simple training program can be done in just *ONE-HOUR!*

* Medical Security Training can, and should be, quite short. A short but intense course can concentrate on basic first-aid principles, and a few specialized pieces of emergency equipment. This equipment should include Narcan (nasal) administration for possible opioid overdose, training in the use of the AED (defibrillator) and CPR. When taught by the right person this can be accomplished in a ONE-hour class!

In this book I'll outline some of the basics. This book is intended as an adjunct to a *Medical Security Team Training Program* from a qualified instructor. The general focus is on *Celebrity* Medical Security, but the information is valuable for others; such as business leaders and various entrepreneurs or other high-profile clients.

As mentioned above, the *Medical Security* training envisioned here should be very brief, and focused on training several specific members designated as part of the *Medical Security Team*. This person(s) should of course be in the immediate proximity of the celebrity at all times, or available immediately and able to respond to their location in **less than two minutes**.

The person or persons in charge of Medical Security would ideally be present at all *events*, but some trained person should also be available near the celebrity 24 hours a day if possible. Wives, husbands, boyfriends, girlfriends, managers, assistants; *anyone* can be trained in Medical Security. Too often, as in the case of drug overdoses, the person is either alone, or with one other person; it is prudent of course to ensure that such individuals alone with the celebrity are always briefed on who to call, and how to call them, in the event of a potential problem.

The principle of *immediate intervention* **without delay** must also be stressed, so that Medical Security can be summoned *immediately* to intervene before it's too late. We cannot forget that the first few minutes of such emergencies are the vital minutes; help must arrive quickly!

The *Medical Security* person should brief all those who will be alone with the celebrity about who to call in the event of a problem, and the fact that that call should be made IMMEDIATELY if *anything* unusual is suspected. It should be made clear that we don't mind a 'false alarm' if it turns out there is no significant problem. If something seems wrong, call Medical Security and 9-1-1.

Although much of the first aid we will discuss here is *basic*, it is basic care that is often the MOST important when it comes to lifesaving in a serious medical emergency. For example, if the victim having a *stroke* is laid down flat, the stroke could be made worse. If a person who has fainted is NOT laid down flat, *that* could make them worse. If someone isn't breathing, we MUST breathe for them, immediately. Too often, if *all* we do is call 9-1-1, the person may die. Sometimes something simple like knowing whether to sit someone up, or lay them down, or roll them on their side can mean the difference between life and death. The first aid intervention we will discuss here is often simple, but vitally important to know.

This training in most procedures is generally *simple first aid*, such as when to sit someone up, when to lay them down, or when to turn them on their side. But we will also discuss the use of several more *advanced* devices and supplies. Several of these first aid items go beyond your typical 'First Aid' course. Some of this equipment is typically taught at the EMT level of training, and medication administration, such as *Narcan*, is usually limited to those with EMT or *Paramedic* training. Although much of this *Medical Security Team Training* is quite basic, some of it also covers more advanced topics.

Other than dressings and bandages, the following list includes the *advanced* first aid supplies recommended to be immediately available, and that the Medical Security Team should be trained to use. A small Medical Security Team Emergency Response bag should contain:

1. A **Bag-Mask-Device** to give rescue breathing to someone struggling to breathe or who has stopped breathing.
2. **Narcan/Naloxone*, nasal spray, to counteract the effects of narcotics (opioids.)
3. Dressing and Bandaging material for serious bleeding; including a **Tourniquet**.

An AED is vital in the event of cardiac arrest!
4. **AED** (Automated External Defibrillator)

Note: An AED is an important life-saving piece of equipment. It is recommended that an AED be part of the Medical Security Team's supplies. These devices typically cost about $2,000!. *Medical Security Training* should include the operation of an AED. Although some venues will have an AED somewhere on site, getting that AED to your location in an emergency may not occur quickly enough. The AED is used to stop *Ventricular Fibrillation* (which is the abnormal heart rhythm that usually occurs causing cardiac arrest.) To have the best chance of reversing this fibrillation <u>the AED must be used within the *first few minutes* following the cardiac arrest</u>. The only way to ensure that the defibrillator will be there soon enough, is to *have one* as part of your Medical Security Team's equipment. *(The fire department, EMT's, or Paramedics will arrive with a defibrillator, but it is typical that their response time will be too long for the defibrillator to be most effective.)*

For every minute that goes by that the heart is not defibrillated, there is a 10% less chance that defibrillation will work. If the 9-1-1 response time is seven minutes for example, there is a 70% chance that the defibrillator will *not* be effective! This means the person will remain in ventricular fibrillation and will ultimately die. ***The Medical Security Team should have their own defibrillator!***

<u>**#2 of the preceding list mentioned *Narcan.***</u> Narcotics, or drugs made from Opiate derivatives, are not limited to Heroin or other *street drugs.* ***Common opioids: Hydrocodone, Methadone, Vicodin, Demerol, Lorcet, OxyContin, Fentanyl.*** Accidental overdose from *prescribed* opioids is all too common. Regardless of how the person may have overdosed, and whether it is from a 'street drug' or a prescribed medication, *Narcan/Naloxone,* can reverse the respiratory depressive effects and allow for the return of normal breathing.

*The following information is from: http://stopoverdoseil.org/narcan.html

What is Narcan™ (naloxone)?

Narcan™ (naloxone) is an opiate antidote. Opioids include heroin and prescription pain pills like morphine, codeine, oxycodone, methadone and Vicodin. When a person is overdosing on an opioid, breathing can slow down or stop and it can very hard to wake them from this state. Narcan™ (naloxone) is a prescription medicine that blocks the effects of opioids and reverses an overdose. It cannot be used to get a person high. If given to a person who has not taken opioids, it will not have any effect on him or her, since there is no opioid overdose to reverse.

How does Narcan™ (naloxone) work?

If a person has taken opioids and is then given Narcan™ (naloxone), the opioids will be knocked out of the opiate receptors in the brain. Narcan™ (naloxone) can help even if opioids are taken with alcohol or other drugs. After a dose of Narcan™ (naloxone), the person should begin to breathe more normally and it will become easier to wake them. It is very important to give help to an overdosing person right away. Brain damage can occur within only a few minutes of an opioid overdose as the result of a lack of oxygen to the brain. Narcan™ (naloxone) gives concerned helpers a window of opportunity to save a life by providing extra time to call 911 and carry out rescue breathing and first aid until emergency medical help arrives.

How is Narcan™ (naloxone) given to an overdosing person?

Narcan™ (naloxone) can be given by intramuscular (IM) injection - into the muscle of the arm, thigh or buttocks - or with a nasal spray device (into the nose). Nasal spray use is less common, but some large cities in the U.S. use the nasal spray version and it can be prescribed.

How long does Narcan™ (naloxone) take to work?

Narcan™ (naloxone) generally works within about 5 minutes. Repeated doses may be necessary if a person is still showing signs of overdose even after the first dose.

How long does Narcan™ (naloxone) take to wear off?

Narcan™ (naloxone) starts to wear off after about 30 minutes and is mostly gone after about 90 minutes. By this time the body has processed enough of the opioids that the overdosing person is unlikely to stop breathing again. In some cases, such as after taking a massive dose or using long-acting opioids like methadone, the patient might need another Narcan™ (naloxone) dose and longer medical observation. Always watch the person after they receive a Narcan™ (naloxone) dose for signs of continued overdose.

Who can be prescribed Narcan™?
According to the *Overdose Prevention Act*, trained individuals are allowed to possess and administer Narcan™ (naloxone) to a person having an overdose.

The key is that *everyone* in the celebrity's inner circle should have *some* level of training regarding *Medical Security*, and that several of those people should have more in-depth training in the use of specialized techniques and equipment as part of the *Medical Security Team*. In the event of a medical emergency *everyone* should know the basics of first aid and CPR and be trained to quickly summon advanced medical care. Panic and confusion at a time like this often results in delayed care, and ultimately the death of the victim.

~

The Five Key Points
of Immediate Medical Intervention:

1. **Calling 9-1-1 is essential**.

   Calling 9-1-1 IMMEDIATELY is vital. You must get help on the way *first*. After you, or someone you have directed has called 9-1-1 for help, you can return to the victim to offer first aid. *Don't delay calling 9-1-1.* Calling a manager, or a personal physician, or anyone else must happen AFTER the 9-1-1 call has been made, not before! **If we are not *sure* if there is a medical emergency, common sense should allow you to recognize *potential* trouble and call 9-1-1 *just to be safe*.** It **is** serious if someone is not responding normally, has slurred speech, confusion, has complaints such as trouble breathing or unusual pain, has unusual weakness or inability to function in some way, or is in *any type* of unusual distress. The call to 9-1-1 should be made now! **When in doubt as to whether you should call 9-1-1, CALL!** A mistake here can be deadly. If you aren't sure if this is an emergency or not, ***treat it like an emergency*** and call 9-1-1 immediately.

2. Being informed, being aware.

During the 9-1-1 call the dispatcher will ask for information. They'll want to know what condition the victim is in, and they'll want to know what happened. Tell them what you know. They'll want to confirm the address and your exact location at that address. Everyone in the celebrity inner circle should know where they are at all times; the name of the location, the room number, and hopefully the address. **Tell the dispatcher the celebrity's name!** Their celebrity status can't hurt. <u>Stay on the phone with the dispatcher unless they tell you to hang up</u>. Do not get frustrated with all the questions they ask, they have most likely *already* dispatched help to your location even though they continue to gather more information. Talking to the dispatcher is NOT delaying the 9-1-1 response. *Be calm, clear, and professional, and give them all the information you know about the situation.*

3. **<u>You</u> are taking charge, YOU must act.**

As part of the celebrity *inner circle* you may or may not be used to being in charge. As a trained member of the *Medical Security Team*, and in the event of a medical emergency, **YOU MUST TAKE CHARGE.** Act quickly, stay calm, and use your training and knowledge to administer appropriate care until professional rescuers take over. After being trained in basic first aid techniques and the use of specialized equipment, you must realize that the application of what you know must be done *quickly*. We cannot wait for someone else to arrive, WE must attempt life-saving care if possible. Time is critical! **We cannot be reluctant to act.** If we have been trained to provide first aid care we must be the one to do it! If the victim isn't breathing, you will use your *Bag Mask Device* to breathe for them. If they are unconscious but breathing, you will turn them on their side (recovery position.) If they have no pulse you will place them on their back on a firm surface and perform CPR. If you believe they may have overdosed on some drug or medication you will administer *Narcan*. You will be trained in what to do, and you must *quickly* do it. The rescuers should be on the way, but they may arrive too late; YOU must act quickly to perform life-saving care.

4. **Don't assume someone is *dead* or that nothing can be done**.

Cardiac arrest, where there is no response, no breathing, and no pulse, can sometimes be reversed; that is what CPR and the defibrillator is for. If you don't have one, the rescuers will arrive with a *defibrillator* that may be able to cause a return of the heartbeat. We should treat the victim that appears to be dead as if they can be resuscitated. We will perform CPR until help arrives and they take over. If the victim is not breathing and has no heartbeat, **the only chance they have to be revived is if YOU quickly perform CPR and use the AED!**

IMPORTANT: If you have a defibrillator you must use that *immediately*, the defibrillator is more important than CPR, it takes priority. If we do nothing but wait for rescuers to arrive, the person will likely die. *We must act quickly to perform CPR and to use an AED if available.*

5. **Plan ahead**.

You must think about various emergency scenarios every day. As part of the *Medical Security Team* you are charged with protecting the life of your employer, and others such as friends and family in the event of a medical emergency. You should remain familiar with all the equipment at your disposal. You should always stay aware of your surroundings and location in case you need to summon help. You should think about potential health and safety risks that may be likely based on your employer's health and habits and the activities they are involved in. As a member of the *Medical Security Team* you will not panic; panic is the result of not knowing what to do, and **you WILL know what to do.** You must act quickly, calmly, and appropriately as a trained member of Medical Security, *that* is your job. During an actual emergency there will be those around you who *do* panic. They may try to do *something*, but it may not be the correct care. As part of a *Medical Security Team* you must take charge, take control, and remain cool. Make sure nobody attempts the *wrong* intervention. Your prompt and proper immediate care and making sure that others do not attempt the *wrong* care, will give those around you the confidence that appropriate first aid is occurring, and this should help to calm others.

~

Your equipment:

1. A ***Bag-Mask-Device*** to give rescue breathing to someone struggling to breathe or who has stopped breathing.
2. *****Narcan**/Naloxone, nasal spray, to counteract the effects of narcotics/opioids.
3. Dressing and **Bandaging** material for serious bleeding; including a ***tourniquet***.
4. **AED** (Automated External Defibrillator)

Those items could be vital during a medical emergency and require specific training to use properly. A first aid kit could also contain other supplies that the Medical Security Team personnel are trained to use, as well as helpful medications such as *Benadryl* for allergic reactions. It is preferable that the first aid kit be simple, that items are easy to see and retrieve, and that only the most important supplies be kept in it.

Let's discuss each of those five items.

1. <u>**A Bag-Mask-Device**</u> **to give rescue breathing to someone struggling to breathe or who has stopped breathing.**

The *Bag-Mask-Device* is a *positive pressure* breathing device, meaning that air is forced into the lungs under pressure when the bag is gently squeezed. It is used when a victim is not breathing, or we suspect that the breathing is not adequate. **WHEN YOU AREN'T SURE THEY ARE BREATHING ADEQUATELY, BREATHE FOR THEM!** *Cyanosis*, or blueness around the lips and face, indicates *severe* lack of oxygen. The Bag-Mask-Device is used instead of mouth-to-mouth breathing to avoid transmission of diseases and to avoid breathing Carbon Dioxide (CO_2) into the victim. <u>**When in doubt as to whether or not breathing is adequate, assist breathing with the Bag-Mask-Device!**</u> We should be worried about a slower than normal respiratory *rate (12-20 times a minute is considered a <u>normal</u> breathing rate)* and, if we believe the victim's **tidal volume** *(the amount of air* *moving in and out of the lungs)* is too shallow, we should assist breathing with the Bag-Mask-Device. *If you suspect breathing is not adequate, assist their breathing.* If the victim *is* breathing, but not adequately, we can simply squeeze the bag as they take a breath in, to make sure the tidal volume is adequate, and their lungs inflate fully. If the rate is too slow, we can add a breath along with their own breathing to increase their rate to 12 breaths per minute. If they are not breathing at all, give about 12 breathes per minute, which is about <u>one breath every five seconds</u>. It is not harmful if we give slightly more breaths per minute. When you are trained in the use of the Bag-Mask-Device you will learn how to place the mask against the face properly, pushing it firmly to make a seal, then tilt the head back correctly, and squeeze the bag *slowly* to administer the breath. *If the bag is squeezed too hard or too fast it could force air into the victim's stomach and cause vomiting.*

Breathing for the victim buys them time for more advanced treatment from professional rescuers and physicians. If breathing stops, for only a few minutes, it can lead to brain damage, and/or cardiac arrest.

<u>**Note:**</u> *If you don't have a Bag-Mask-Device, you could do* <u>*mouth-to-mouth breathing*</u> *for the victim,* ***using an approved barrier device.*** *You would pinch the nose, then seal your lips around theirs and give a breath, just until the chest rises. Medical Security should have a Bag-Mask-Device!*

<u>**Note about vomiting:**</u> If vomit or other fluid is in the mouth, we should also place the victim *on their side*

(recovery position) to allow fluid to drain out and not collect at the back of the throat near their airway (trachea.) Any time a victim vomits they should be *immediately* turned on their side. *Any victim who is confused or not fully conscious should be placed on their side and kept on their side.*

2. <u>**Dressing and Bandaging material**</u>**, for serious bleeding, and the use of a tourniquet.**

Part of your training as a Medical Security Team member should include the proper application of dressings and bandages to cover wounds or to stop serious bleeding, along with other procedures used to stop or slow down bleeding. *A "dressing" is what we place next to the wound, the "bandage" is what holds the dressing in place.*

"Direct Pressure" applied FIRMLY and CONTINUOUSLY should stop most bleeding. A tourniquet is usually not needed, since most serious bleeding can be controlled with firm direct pressure on the wound. <u>But, if firm direct pressure does not quickly control the bleeding, and it is heavy bleeding, use a tourniquet.</u>

(A tourniquet is used for life-threatening bleeding on extremities, arms and legs.) **Part of your training should include the use of a tourniquet.**

As *Medical Security*, when it comes to dressings and bandaging, our focus is *life-threatening* situations, not necessarily Band-Aids on scratches. Although there's nothing wrong with a few Band-Aids in your Medical Response bag.

3. *Narcan/Naloxone, nasal spray to counteract the effects of narcotics.

We mentioned this medication earlier, and detailed it uses. *Narcan* is effective with medications/drugs that are *opiate* derivatives. Too many of the deaths listed at the beginning of this book involved narcotic (opiate) drugs or medications that depress breathing. Opioid overdose is an epidemic in the United States! The risk of such substances is primarily their *respiratory depressant* effects. The victim dies because their breathing slows down, and then stops. Many prescription medications can cause such adverse reactions, especially those used for sleep or pain, and such medications are COMMON. Although Heroin is a big offender when it comes to respiratory depression and death, other common narcotics are morphine, codeine, hydrocodone. oxycodone, methadone and Vicodin.

Although *Narcan* is not effective for barbiturates, we should be aware that this same respiratory depressant effect can occur with barbiturates. Some of the more common barbiturates are, phenobarbital, amobarbital (Amytal), pentobarbital (Nembutal), and secobarbital (Seconal).

Note: Judy Garland, and Jimi Hendrix, died from barbiturate overdose.

4. AED (Automated External Defibrillator)

As part of *Medical Security Team* Training you should learn to operate an AED. The AED is **only** attached to a victim if they are unresponsive, not breathing, and have no pulse; you would also begin CPR on this victim. If your equipment does not include an AED, you would immediately ask if the venue or location you are at has one. After you are trained in the operation of the AED *you ARE allowed to use any available AED in the event of an emergency.*

Many things could cause a cardiac arrest; heart attack, drug overdose, drowning, electric shock, even dieting that disrupts the levels of potassium or causes other imbalances of vital minerals and electrolytes in the body. In cardiac arrest the heart is most often in *Ventricular Fibrillation,* which causes the heart to stop pumping and just *quiver.* In Ventricular Fibrillation the victim will NOT have a pulse. The AED delivers a shock that *stops* this fibrillation. A defibrillator is **not** a 'jump start' to the heart like a car battery. After the AED has wiped out the fibrillation, our hope is that the heart is not too severely damaged, and that the pacemaker cells in the heart begin to send out electrical pulses, and that the heart begins to beat again.

The AED has an electronic voice and very few buttons or controls, and it tells you what to do. The adhesive electrode patches that attach to the chest have illustrations, showing where each of the two patches should be placed on the chest. *(Some AED's have <u>one large patch</u>, with a picture that shows you how to place it on the chest.)* During your Medical Security training you should learn about the specific functions of the AED you will use, and the general rules for all AED's. Most AED's are quite similar, and even if you must use an AED different than the one you were trained on, it will be simple to use, and you can use it!

When needed, the AED must be used within the *first few minutes* of a cardiac arrest to be effective!

* ALL Medical Security Teams SHOULD HAVE AN AED as part of their emergency response kit.

NOTE: *Some AEDs will monitor the CPR being given and will remind you to push harder if needed or to speed up or slow down your compressions.* **You should have a more advanced AED that will assist and guide you with proper CPR compressions.**

Other medical problems:

We talked earlier about the use of *Narcan* for opiate drug overdose. It is important to note that the victim does not necessarily have to be a chronic drug abuser to suffer a negative consequence or be at risk. Potentially dangerous medications can be introduced following a medical procedure, injury, or illness. The potential for an accidental overdose, or serious negative reaction to the medication, is always a concern. Even *alcohol* can be a killer.

This information is from *The National Institute on Alcohol abuse and Alcoholism*

http://pubs.niaaa.nih.gov/publications/AlcoholOverdoseFactsheet/Overdosefact.htm

Continuing to drink despite clear signs of significant impairments can result in a potentially deadly type of overdose called alcohol poisoning.

Alcohol poisoning occurs when there is so much alcohol in the bloodstream that areas of the brain controlling basic

life-support functions—such as breathing, heart rate, and temperature control—begin to shut down. Symptoms of alcohol poisoning include confusion; difficulty remaining conscious; vomiting; seizures; trouble with breathing; slow heart rate; clammy skin; dulled responses, such as no gag reflex (which prevents choking); and extremely low body temperature.

BAC (Blood Alcohol Content) can continue to rise even when a person is unconscious. Alcohol in the stomach and intestine continues to enter the bloodstream and circulate throughout the body.

It is dangerous to assume that an unconscious person will be fine by sleeping it off. Alcohol acts as a depressant, hindering signals in the brain that control automatic responses such as the gag reflex. Alcohol also can irritate the stomach, causing vomiting. With no gag reflex, a person who drinks to the point of passing out is in danger of choking on vomit, which, in turn, could lead to death by asphyxiation. Even if the drinker survives, an alcohol overdose can lead to long-lasting brain damage.

What Should I Do If I Suspect Someone Has Alcohol Poisoning?

- Know the danger signals
- Do not wait for someone to have all the symptoms
- Be aware that a person who has passed out may die
- *If you suspect an alcohol overdose, call 911 for help*

What Can Happen to Someone with Alcohol Poisoning That Goes Untreated?

- Choking on his or her own vomit

- Breathing that slows, becomes irregular, or stops
- Heart that beats irregularly or stops
- Hypothermia (low body temperature)
- Hypoglycemia (too little blood sugar), which leads to seizures
- Untreated severe dehydration from vomiting, which can cause seizures, permanent brain damage, and death

*If you suspect someone has alcohol poisoning, get medical help immediately. Cold showers, hot coffee, or walking **will not** reverse the effects of alcohol overdose and could actually make things worse.*

Of course, there are *many* illnesses, injuries, and potential medical complications that could occur. As part of a *Medical Security Team* we probably aren't doctors, or certified EMT's or licensed Paramedics, but we are trained in the basics of first aid, CPR, and the use of special equipment, and we do have knowledge about what to do that many around us do not have.

We should be familiar with the most common medical problems we might encounter. We will discuss those specific problems in the next chapter.

Note:

If the person who you are providing Medical Security for has any specific medical conditions or concerns; such as allergies, or special medical devices such as a pacemaker or implanted defibrillator, or if they have a known substance abuse issue, you should be aware of this, and in some cases (such as diabetes, or allergies) you should carry special supplies appropriate for the illness, such as *glucose paste for diabetes*, or an *EpiPen* for allergic reactions, and, make sure you understand how to administer these items.

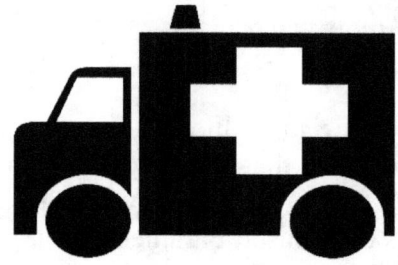

Chapter Three

COMMON MEDICAL PROBLEMS

The essential first aid
for various medical problems:

*We should always try to think of the most serious condition that may be occurring (the worst-case scenario) and treat the victim as if they have **that** problem. It is much safer to over-treat than to under-treat.*

Difficulty breathing.

Many things can cause breathing troubles; heart disease, lung disease, allergic reactions, drug overdose, blot clots, choking, just to name a few. All of these problems will require the attention of a doctor. When breathing problems are severe it is obvious that the victim needs medical help, but if the problem is minor, or just beginning, the victim may wait it out, or try some over-the-counter remedy, but that is a *mistake*. Even the most minor complaint of difficulty breathing should be considered an emergency, and 9-1-1 should be called right away. Any *noisy* breathing is a sign of trouble. Some heart conditions, and other medical problems, can cause *wet sounding* breathing from fluid in the lungs; THAT is also an emergency! Breathing problems, even if it seems minor, are emergencies! Our first aid for breathing problems is limited.

Keep the person sitting up. If we had oxygen, that might help some, but would not be a cure. If the problem is caused from an allergic reaction *Benadryl* may help, but that should not take the place of calling 9-1-1 and getting professional help. If the airways leading to the lungs close down from inflammation, as in an allergic reaction, smoke inhalation, or Asthma, the victim may make a wheezing sound as they breathe, and the victim can die without medical attention. Our first aid for severe Asthma would include **keeping the person sitting up** and assisting the ventilations with a Bag-Mask-Device if they are not moving sufficient air on their own. <u>If the person whose breathing we are assisting becomes unconscious, we should then lay them down and continue assisting their breathing</u>, making sure they have at least one breath every five seconds. If the chest does not seem to rise properly with each breath, or we suspect that there is some sort of *obstruction* in the airway, we have two choices; if we think there may be swelling in the mouth, or that the tongue may be blocking the airway, we can tilt the head back, which should move the tongue and open the airway. *Some AED's use the AED lid, placed under the victim's upper back, to help to keep the head tilted back.* The other possibility is a *foreign body* in the airway, this is something that doesn't belong in the airway that we must attempt to remove. If the person has choked on some object, we can use choking procedures like the *Heimlich maneuver* to try to get it out. Your training books will discuss these specific options.

Chest pain.

We should always think of the worst-case when it comes to medical complaints, and <u>it's always best to over-treat than to under-treat the victim</u>. When it comes to *chest pain*, we should consider the possibility of a *heart attack*. A heart

34

attack, or *Myocardial Infarction*, is the result of the death (infarction) of some portion of the heart (the myocardium.) *Infarction* means dead tissue. When this occurs in the heart, it can affect the heart's ability to pump blood, may disrupt the normal rhythmic heartbeat, and can cause the heart to fibrillate (quiver instead of pump) which will result in cardiac arrest (no breathing, no heartbeat) which requires CPR and the quick application of a defibrillator, if the victim is to have any chance of survival.

Chest pain, which may be the sign of a heart attack in progress, or the warning sign of impending heart damage from lack of oxygen to the heart, is a serious complaint. We must call 9-1-1 immediately and **lay the person flat**. If they are pale or sweaty, we should also elevate their legs about 18 inches (shock position.) If they become unconscious, we must check their breathing and pulse. If they are unresponsive and there is no breathing and no pulse, begin CPR and apply the AED. Your training as part of the *Medical Security Team* will include CPR. Your training may concentrate on adult "Hands Only" CPR, or might include choking procedures for Adults, Children, and Infants. The *American Heart Association*® offers CPR classes to allow for more practice with manikins, and to obtain CPR and Choking training for children and infants if not covered in your Medical Security Course.

Unconsciousness.

When a person becomes unresponsive to your voice, and will not respond, or responds to tapping their shoulder firmly by only moaning or mumbling, the patient is unconscious. There is a risk when a person is unconscious that they will not be able to control their airway and may choke if they vomit. Any time a person is unconscious, or very confused and lethargic (sleepy) **we should place them in *recovery position* (on their side.)** We should also call 9-1-1. Even if this condition is caused from alcohol, it can be serious. Letting the person 'sleep it off' is a dangerous choice. Consider tilting the head back if there is noisy breathing (snoring sounds) and monitor their breathing and prepare to use the Bag-Mask-Device if breathing becomes weak or labored. Monitor their pulse and begin CPR and use the AED if they stop breathing and have no pulse.

If we aren't <u>SURE</u> as to whether they have a pulse, or whether they are breathing, we should start CPR!

* Studies have shown that checking for a pulse can be difficult, and that many people are not SURE if they feel a pulse or not. If you are not SURE you feel a pulse, and they show no signs of movement or breathing, start CPR. If you aren't SURE they are breathing, and they have no other signs of life, start CPR.

Seizure.

A person who has *epilepsy* (seizure disorder) may take medications to attempt to reduce the possibility of having seizures but may have seizures from time to time despite their medication. A seizure may also result from an overdose, stroke, head injury, brain tumor, and other causes. The main type of seizure is a *grand mal seizure*, which causes the person to become unconscious and causes full-body contractions. We should call 9-1-1 whenever a person has a seizure. Most often the seizure activity will be short, less than a minute, and is usually followed by a period of sleepiness and confusion (the *post ictal* period.) During the seizure activity we should **not** try to hold the person down or stop the shaking, and we should **NOT** put *anything* into their mouth. Vomiting is not that common while seizing, but we can **roll the person to their side during the seizure to better protect their airway**. After the seizure, during the post ictal period, which can be short or may last for several minutes, we are NOT in a hurry to wake them up. As long as they are breathing adequately, we should leave them alone. People often worry about the person *biting their tongue*, or, wrongly, *swallowing* their tongue (you can't swallow your tongue.) If the person does bite their tongue during the seizure it is usually a minor injury, usually requiring no special care to heal. Because of the danger of putting objects into the mouth, and the fact that if they do bite their tongue it has probably already happened, **we *never* put objects into a person's mouth during or after a seizure.** A seizure is potentially a serious problem and requires an immediate call to 9-1-1.

Confusion.

This is a warning sign. Whatever the reason, if a person becomes confused, we should call 9-1-1 and have them examined by a doctor. Confusion could be the first sign of an overdose on drugs, alcohol, or medication. It could be the result of a stroke, or low or high blood pressure, diabetic conditions involving high or low blood sugar, and many other causes. There are many reasons why a person may become confused, and most are serious. Whatever the reason, becoming confused is a sign of a potentially serious medical problem. Unless we see signs of a *stroke*, **when someone is confused, we should lay them down and put their feet up** in *shock position.* Shock position will cause blood to move to the brain, which may improve the person's condition somewhat, especially if their condition is the result of low blood pressure. *If they seem to have signs of a stroke, keep them sitting up, using shock position for a stroke victim could make the stroke worse!*

Stroke.

Cerebral Vascular Accident, or CVA, is the medical term for a stroke. A stroke is a brain problem and is caused either by bleeding in the brain from a burst vessel, or a blood clot plugging a vessel in the brain. Either of these situations will reduce the blood flow to some part of the brain, usually causing damage, often permanent damage, to that portion of the brain. Strokes often cause signs such as one-sided weakness or paralysis, slurred speech, confusion, headache, blurred vision, loss of bowel or bladder control, or unconsciousness. A stroke can result in death. Often, but not always, a stroke is related to high blood pressure. Because of the link between stroke and high blood pressure **it is usually best to keep the victim with signs of a stroke *sitting up*.** As we mentioned previously, under the *confusion* section, if we put a stroke victim in shock position we might make the stroke even worse, by causing more pressure, and more bleeding in the brain. If we kept someone sitting up for any reason, but *then* they *become* unconscious, we should then lay them down.

Bleeding.

Bleeding, even serious bleeding like an amputation, is usually easily controlled with *direct pressure* on the site of the bleeding. Bleeding from cut *veins* (venous bleeding) is usually a steady bleed, and not as serious as *arterial* bleeding which spurts blood from an artery with each beat of the heart. Venous bleeding is usually well-controlled with a simple dressing and light pressure over the wound. Regardless of the type of bleeding, direct pressure should stop it. It would be best to use latex type gloves to avoid contact with blood, and some sort of *dressing* to place on top of the cut, and then our gloved hand to apply pressure over the dressing. The pressure may need to be *significant*, especially to control *arterial* bleeding. <u>If the dressing soaks through, don't remove it, place another dressing over it and apply MORE pressure.</u> **Once we have controlled the bleeding with direct pressure we should *continue* applying the firm pressure until other medical personnel take over.** During training as a *Medical Security Team* member, you will also learn other methods to control bleeding, such as the use of a *tourniquet*.

Other concerns.

Shootings, terrorism, burns, explosions, car accidents, etc. The list of potential emergencies is extensive, and our emergency care is often limited. We must remember that first aid from minimally trained bystanders or even from more extensively trained Medical Security is often limited to a few specific first aid principles:

Difficulty breathing: Keep the person sitting up. *(If they become unconscious lay them down, check pulse and breathing.)*

Chest pain: Lay the person down in 'shock position.'

Unconscious: Lay the person on their side in 'recovery position.'

Seizure: Leave them alone. After the seizure, place them on their side in 'recovery position.'

Confusion: Lay the person down in 'shock position.'

Stroke: Keep the person sitting up. *(If they become unconscious lay them down, check pulse and breathing.)*

Bleeding: Apply and maintain direct pressure, or a tourniquet if needed.

CPR: Perform 'chest compressions' any time the person has no breathing and no pulse or if you are *unsure* they are breathing and have a pulse. When in doubt, do CPR!

With "Hands Only" CPR, where you give **no** breaths, and simply push on the chest, you will cause air to move in and out of the lungs with each chest compression. If you have a Bag-Mask-Device and are confident in how to use it, CPR would include 30 chest compressions followed by 2 breaths with the Bag-Mask. If you do not have a Bag-Mask-Device, or are not familiar with more advanced CPR, "Hands Only" CPR with no breaths is perfectly fine. Remember, you will be causing "breathing" with each chest compression as air is forced out and is then passively pulled back in.

Note:

For gunshot injuries.

Our main concern is bleeding. We should be able to control *external* bleeding with our bandaging materials and direct pressure on the wound. We will be familiar with the use of a tourniquet if bleeding on an extremity cannot be controlled with direct pressure.

But with a gunshot wound to the torso, the problem is most likely *internal* bleeding. We have no good treatment for internal bleeding. The person needs to have emergency surgery immediately and we must make sure 9-1-1 has been called to transport them.

Our first aid will likely be limited to pressure on bleeding wounds, perhaps a tourniquet, and assistance with their airway, breathing and/or CPR if needed.

Anyone who looks "shocky," pale, cool, sweaty; lay them down, and elevate their feet 12-18 inches.

Chapter Four

Medical Security Team Training

IF WE KNOW WHAT TO DO, WE WON'T PANIC

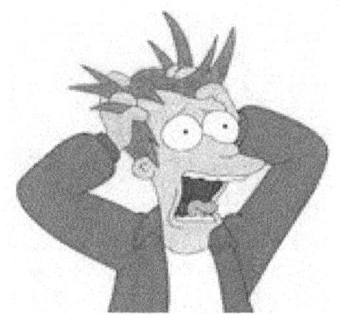

The essential training for *Medical Security Team* personnel is significant but can be accomplished in just one-hour! A long and complicated training course is often not advised, because it is sometimes difficult to fit such training into the busy schedule of one's employees, and because too much information will be more difficult to retain. Because our intervention is limited to a few specific actions, and training in only a few specific pieces of equipment, we can make *Medical Security Team Training* brief. **Training in Medical Security must, in my opinion, cover the following essential topics:**

1. Training in recognition of medical emergencies. Calling 9-1-1 and our interaction with the 9-1-1 operator. Discussion of the duties of the Medical Security Team.

2. CPR *may be limited to "Adult Hands Only CPR"* or might include instruction on Children and Infants CPR and Choking procedures. MUST INCLUDE INSTRUCTION ON THE USE OF THE AED!

3. An introduction to common medical problems to include:

    a. Difficulty breathing
    b. Chest pain
    c. Unconsciousness/OD
    d. Seizures
    e. Confusion
    f. Stroke
    g. Bleeding

4. The use of important first aid equipment to include:

    a. Bag-Mask-Device device
    b. Dressings, bandages, tourniquets
    c. Narcan/Naloxone
    d. AED

The training course should include scenario practice to test the application of proper response procedures, the proper use of all first aid equipment, and practice with these devices on a manikin. The course should also include individual practice in CPR on CPR manikins.

Class size should be limited to approximately (5) people at a time, to insure proper one-on-one attention and to maximize the supervision of skills practice.

Medical Security Team Training should be renewed *annually*, with the entire course repeated. Remember, this course can be completed in as little as **ONE HOUR**, which is what makes this training unique, and which makes annual renewal more likely to take place.

It is recommended that all those within the client's *inner circle* have this training. **At a minimum there should always be at least one person with this level of training available in the immediate vicinity *(available within two minutes)* of the client.**

It is also important that the person doing this training has real-world experience in emergency medical care, preferably as an emergency responder in a *busy* jurisdiction. **I believe that the trainer should be an EMT or Paramedic.** I'm prejudiced here, but an EMT or Paramedic will probably make a better teacher of this level of medical care than would a doctor! The doctor's expertise is in the *hospital* setting, and a doctor tends to teach too many *details* that are not important with this level of care. The EMT and Paramedic's expertise is in *pre-hospital* care, which is where these emergencies will occur. The Medical Security Team instructor should have *experience as an instructor;* a good EMT, Paramedic or Firefighter/Paramedic is not *necessarily* a good teacher.

The concept of *Medical Security* is important. In the event of a medical emergency having staff with this training could be a matter of life and death.

When I review the list of celebrities who have died and realize that some whose deaths may have been prevented, the importance of this training hits home.

Those of you who obtain such *Medical Security Team* training have a heavy responsibility. You are charged with quickly and appropriately responding to offer potential life-saving care. You are expected to act calmly and professionally and to be well-trained in basic first aid skills and several more advanced skills. You are expected to maintain a high level of proficiency in these skills, and to obtain refresher training each year.

It is my hope that this training becomes common-place, and that the term "Medical Security" becomes a norm, and that we can begin to see positive outcomes following a medical emergency, where in the past it has too often been tragically negative.

Lance Hodge

Medical Security

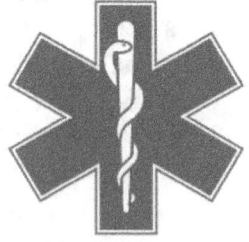

Team

To arrange *Medical Security Team* Training at your location, contact me:

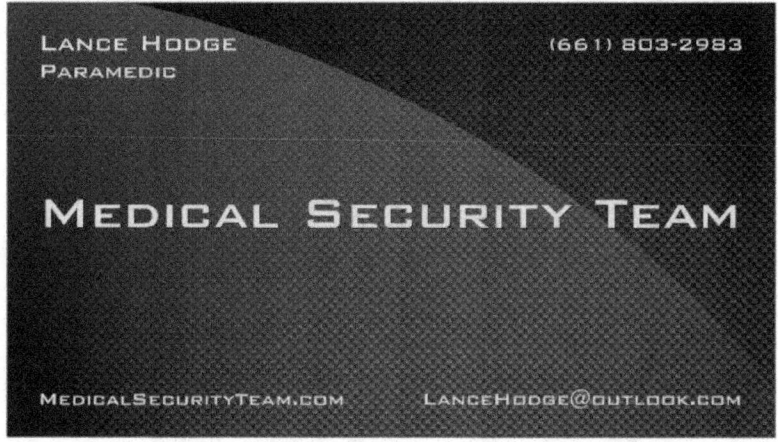

Lance Hodge
LanceHodge@outlook.com

P.S.

*I have a short book on Amazon called **"5-Minute CPR."** That book would be a valuable resource for a Medical Security Training course.*

~

I have another goal; a big idea that hopes to change the paradigm of survival from cardiac arrest. Fifty years ago, before our Paramedic programs were created, only 5% of people in cardiac arrest could be saved. Now, fifty years later, the save rate for those in cardiac arrest outside of hospitals, is **still** about 5%.

Something has gone wrong.

The problem; people don't know how to do CPR and, most importantly, _AED's don't get to these people in time._

Thousands of lives could be saved every year if new homes being built came *with* an AED! My book, **"An AED at Home"** attempts to get home builders interested in this concept of placing an AED in their new home projects.

Of the 350,000 cardiac arrests that occur each year, 80% occur at HOME!

~

More information, contact me at:
LanceHodge@outlook.com